Homemade Household Cleaners

40 Recipes of Safe Cleaners for Tiles, Stoves, Ovens and Kitchen Countertops

Table of Contents

Introduction

Safety cleaners have always been a cause of concern for people who are too conscious about their health. The problem always arises because of the supermarket safety cleaners consisting of a lot of chemicals along with being extremely expensive.

Recently, a few cases related to causing cancer, asthma and migraine were reported which cause a great hue. People now feel much better to make their safety cleaners at their homes rather than buy the readily made ones.

Making safety cleaners at home is no hard work and requires just a few ingredients which can make up to great solutions and perform the same kind of work which the ready made ones do.

The difference is only the texture and the packaging. Apart from that, safety cleaners that are made at home neither contain chemicals nor do they involve a lot of expense at your cause.

With the help of this amazing book, here is a great opportunity for you to learn 40 instant recipes of safety cleaners that you can read, understand and then make them at your home.

These recipes are simple and quickly made, and you can then use them either on your tiles, ovens, oven burners, kitchen counter tops or to clean your windows.

So, get this book as fast as you can and tell it to your friends and families as well. Unite together in to not buying the supermarket safety cleaners for good health and focus on making these homemade safety cleaners which are not only cheap to make but also not that dangerous!

Recipe 01: All-purpose cleaner

Description: Kill germs in your kitchen and on your bathroom tiles with this all-purpose cleaner which can be made so cheaply as compared to those available in the markets.

Ingredients:

- Water- 2 cups
- Vinegar- 4 tablespoons
- Spray bottle- 1

Directions:

- With the help of a spray bottle, add in the cups of water.
- Next add in the vinegar.
- Shake to mix both the ingredients.
- Spray on any dirty surface such as kitchen counter tops and then clean away with a damp towel.

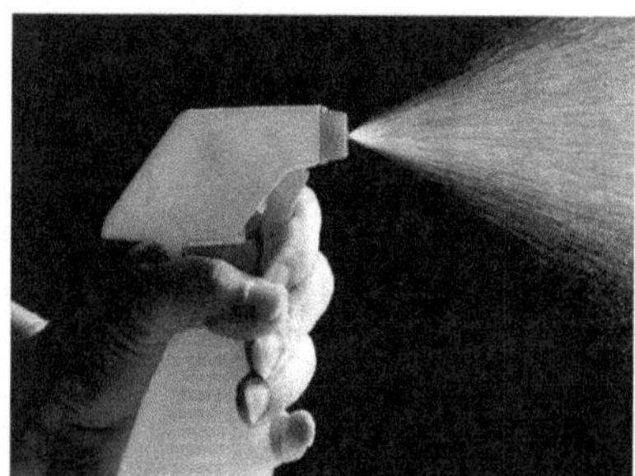

Recipe 02: Tile cleaner

Description: The tile cleaners readily available in the markets consist of a lot of contaminants and chemicals associated with causing cancer. It is better to make your own tile cleaner at home.

Ingredients:

- Baking soda- ½ cup
- Liquid soap- ½ cup
- Lavender essential oil- 5 drops
- Tea tree oil- 5 drops

Directions:

- Take a bowl and add in the baking soda.
- Mix in the liquid soap until the mixture becomes frothy.
- Now mix in the lavender essential oil and the tea tree essential oil.
- Put this mixture on your sponge and scrub the desired place which needs to be cleaned.

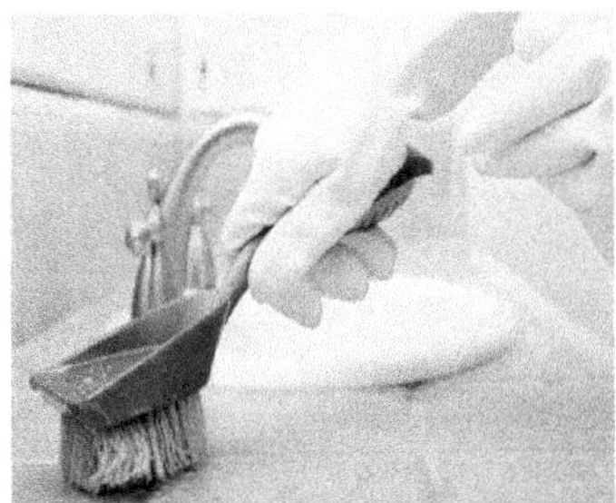

Recipe 03: The best oven cleaner recipe

Description: The oven cleaners that are available in the super markets have a lot of harsh ingredients which cause pollution in the air. It is better to make this oven cleaner at home as this recipe works really well.

Ingredients:

- Hot water- 2 cups
- Dishwashing liquid- 1 tablespoon
- Borax- 1 teaspoon

Directions:

- Take a bowl and add in the hot water.
- Now mix in the dishwashing liquid.
- Next add in the borax and mix well.
- Pour this mixture in to a spray bottle and shake to mix.
- Spray this on your oven and let it stay there for 20 to 25 minutes.
- Wipe the dirt now with a clean cloth.

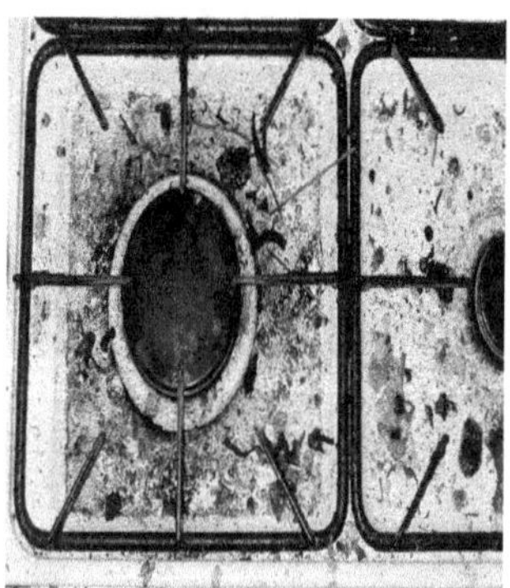

Recipe 04: Window cleaner

Description: Make this homemade window cleaner which will prevent allergies and asthma from accumulating just like the ones from the supermarket do.

Ingredients:

- Vinegar- ¼ cup
- Dishwashing liquid- ½ teaspoon
- Water- 2 cups

Directions:

- Put the vinegar, dishwashing liquid and the water in to a spray bottle and mix to shake.
- Spray this on the window glass and scrub with a sponge.
- Wipe off with first a wet cloth and then with a dry cotton cloth.
- Put your wiping clothes in the washing machine and enjoy your clean and sparkling windows.

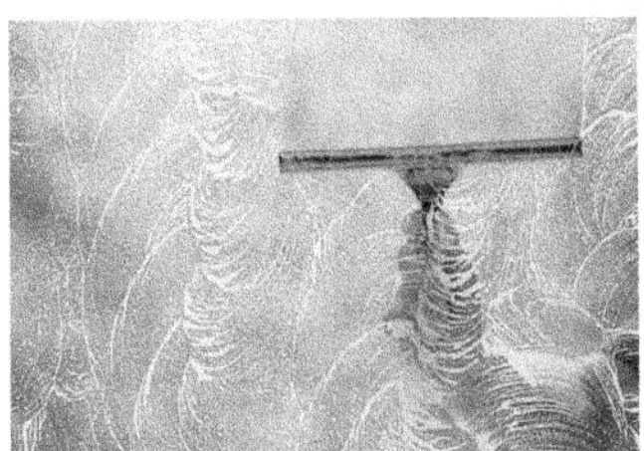

Recipe 05: Lemon oil duster

Description: There is a lot of dust at our homes and it is loaded with flame retardants, pesticides and chemicals. The dust cleaners available in the supermarkets might have traces of air contaminants which is why it is advised to make this duster at home.

Ingredients:

- Lemon oil- 10 drops
- Lemon juice- 2 tablespoons
- Olive oil- 5 drops

Directions:

- Take a spray bottle and add in the lemon oil drops.
- Now add in the lemon juice and the olive oil.
- Mix the spray bottle to mix together the ingredients.
- Spray on dusty surfaces and then wipe off with a damp towel.

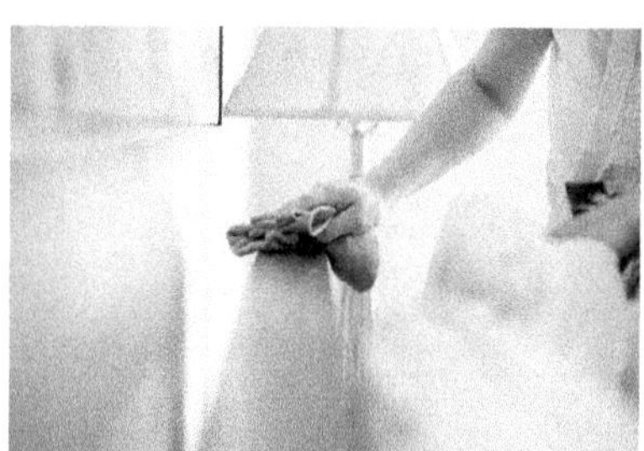

Recipe 06: Multi- surface cleaner

Description: This multi-surface cleaner is a great way to clean your surfaces and the best solution to prevent your crawling babies from getting germs and bacteria from the floor.

Ingredients:

- Borax- 2 teaspoons
- Washing soda- 1 teaspoon
- Hot water- 2 cups
- Vinegar- 4 tablespoons
- Natural liquid soap- ½ teaspoon
- Tea tree oil- ¼ teaspoon
- Rosemary oil- 8 drops
- Tangerine oil- 8 drops
- Lavender essential oil- 8 drops

Directions:

- Add the hot water in a boil and mix together the borax and the washing soda and mix until dissolved.
- Strain the mixture through a sieve to prevent any lumps from accumulating.
- Now mix in the vinegar, natural liquid soap, tea tree oil, rosemary oil, tangerine oil and the lavender essential oil.
- Mix together all the ingredients and pour them in to a spray bottle.
- Spray on to a dirty surface and then clean with a damp towel to clean the mess.

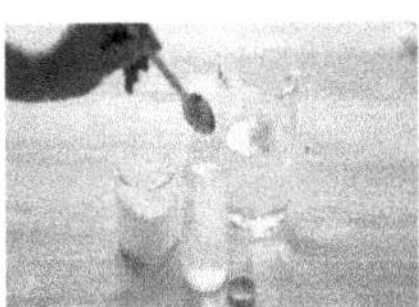

Recipe 07: Laundry powder

Description: There is a great chance that the laundry powders available in the supermarkets have a lot of artificial fragrance which may cause migraine to you and a severe headache. Save your money and health with the help of this laundry powder.

Ingredients:

- Soap flakes- ½ cup
- Borax- ½ cup
- Washing soda- ½ cup

Directions:

- Take a jar and add in the soap flakes.
- Now add in the borax.
- Next add in the washing soda and mix to combine all the ingredients.
- Close the jar and store it and use it when required.

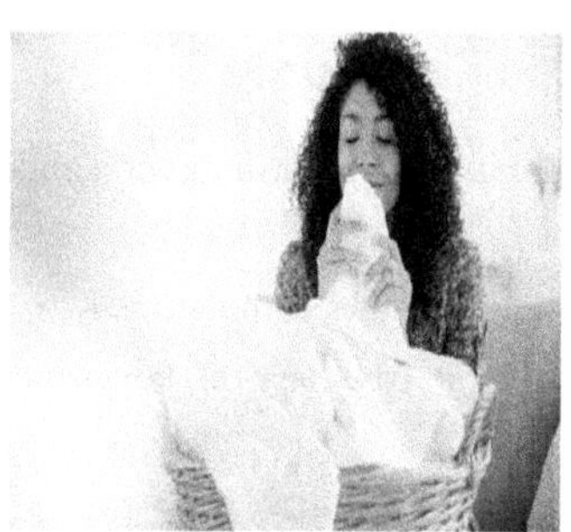

Recipe 08: Tub and sink cleaner

Description: Tubs and sinks tend to get dirty more often as they are used quite regularly. Make this spray cleaner at home and easily clean your bathroom and get amazing results.

Ingredients:

- Vinegar- 1 ½ cups
- Water- 1 ½ cups
- Hydrogen peroxide- ¾ cup
- Lavender essential oil- 6 drops
- Eucalyptus essential oil- 5 drops

Directions:

- Take a spray bottle and add in the vinegar and the water.
- Shake to dissolve.
- Now add in the hydrogen peroxide, lavender essential oil and the eucalyptus essential oil.
- Close the spray bottle and shake to mix together.
- Spray on your tubs and sink and let it stay for 10 minutes before rubbing it with a damp towel.

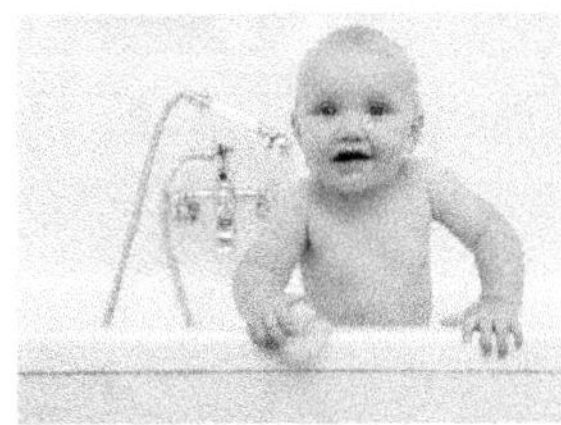

Recipe 09: Light tile cleaners

Description: Use this light tile cleaners to clean your tiles if the dirt is little and light. The dirt will be easily removed with the help of this tile cleaner. The tea tree oil added has anti-bacterial properties which help fight bacterias on the surface.

Ingredients:

- Baking soda- ¾ cup
- Dish soap- ¼ cup
- Water- 2 tablespoons
- Tea tree oil- 5 drops

Directions:

- Combine together the water, baking soda and the dish soap.
- Mix and then add in the tea tree oil.
- Dip in your sponge in this liquid and then on the tiles.
- Let stay a while then clean with a damp towel.

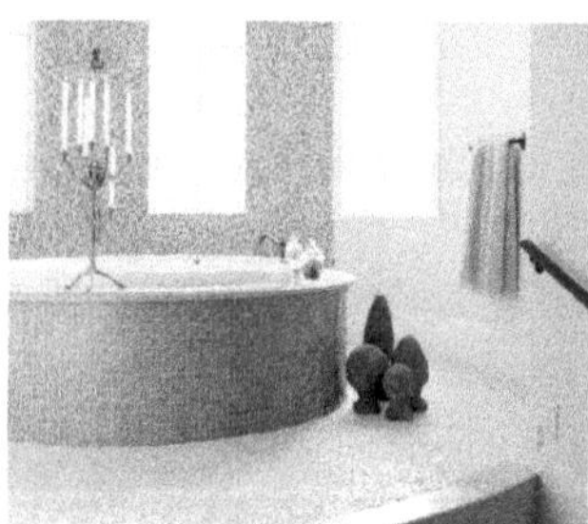

Recipe 10: How to clean your toilet bowl

Description: Toilet bowls tend to get dirty and it is very important to clean them regularly to prevent the growth of bacteria and germs from spreading. Make this easy toilet bowl cleaner using simple ingredients.

Ingredients:

- Borax powder- 2 tablespoons
- Lemon juice, squeezed- 1

Directions:

- Take a lemon and squeeze its juice in to a bowl.
- Now add in the borax powder.
- Mix together both the ingredients until combined.
- Pour this liquid in to your toilet bowl and then scrub it with the help of a brush.
- Flush to remove the dirt.
- Repeat this process every 2 days to get a spotless and clean toilet.

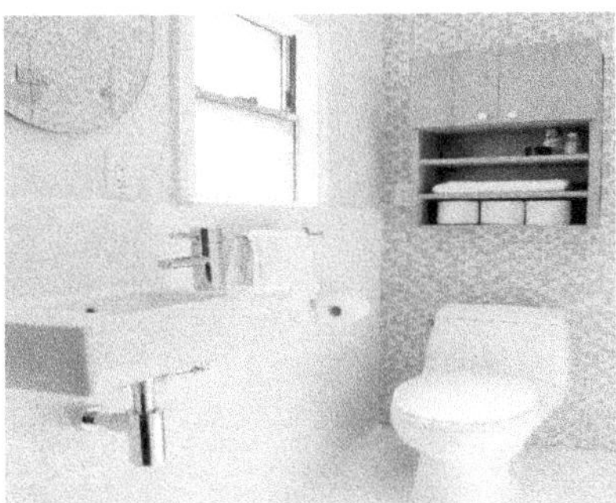

Recipe 11: How to prevent clogging drains

Description: Drains often clog due to big particles trying to go through in and this can be a real problem when you want to use your basin.

Ingredients:

- Baking soda- 1 cup
- White vinegar- 2 cups

Directions:

- Pour the baking soda and the white vinegar in to your clogged basin.
- Open the warm water to let go of the vinegar and baking soda.
- The fizzing and bubbling will finish the clogging and let the water go smoothly.
- This method is also great if your drain is really smelly.

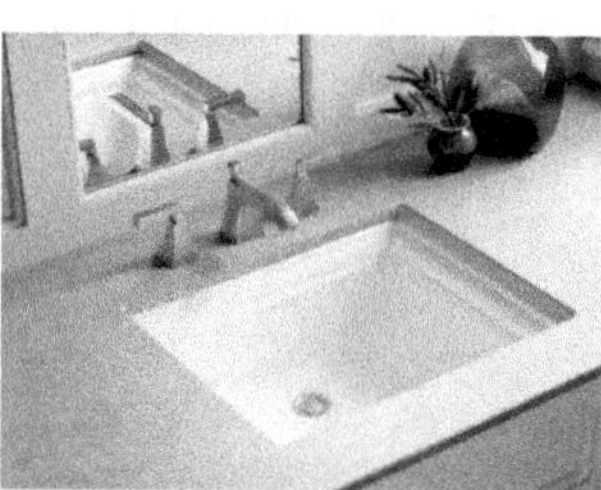

Recipe 12: Shower cleaner

Description: Our showers can sometimes also turn to be greased and dirty. Below is a recipe of a daily shower cleaner which you can use it to clean it well and proper.

Ingredients:

- Distilled water- 1 cup
- White vinegar- 1 cup
- Organic cleaner- 1 ½ teaspoons
- Tea tree essential oil- 10 drops
- Thieves essential oil- 10 to 12 drops

Directions:

- Take the spray bottle and put in the water and the vinegar.
- Then add in the organic cleaner and then add the drops of the tea tree essential oil, and the thieves essential oil.
- Mix it and cover the bottle with the cap.
- After you are done with your shower use the spray to clean.
- Wipe it away with the help of a damp cloth and see the results instantly.

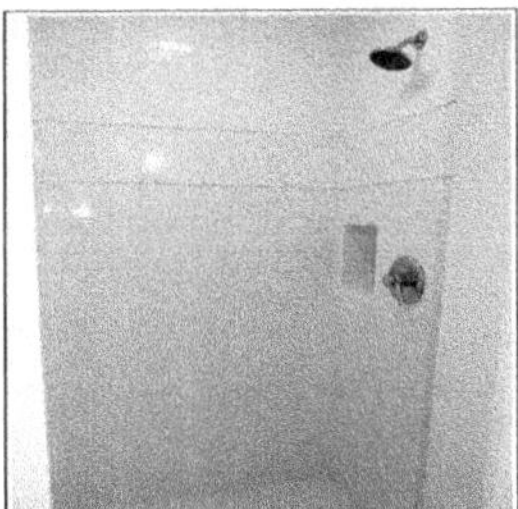

Recipe 13: Natural oven cleaner

Description: All day using of the oven, specially for hard cookers makes the oven often very dirty and greases which are very difficult to remove. Below is a recipe of an oven cleaner with just a few ingredients.

Ingredients:

- Baking soda- ¾ cup
- Orange essential oil- 14 to 15 drops
- Pine essential oil- 15 drops
- Tea tree essential oil- 10 drops
- Water- 3 to 4 tablespoons

Recipe:

- Take a bowl and mix in the water, baking soda, pine essential oil, tea tree essential oil, and orange essential oil and mix it till it forms a paste.
- Apply the mixture to the affected areas of the oven and after few minutes clean it with a sponge.
- The dirt should be now removed.

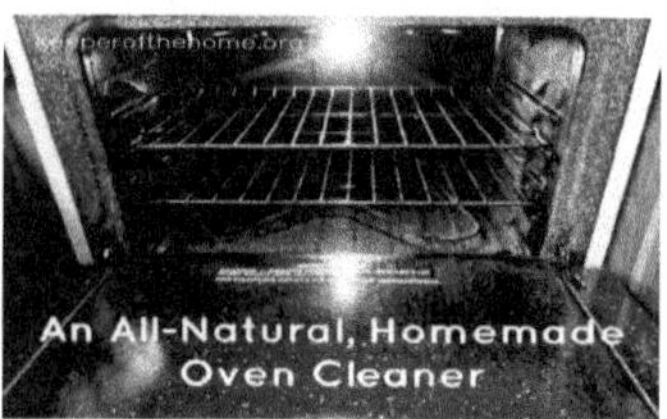

Recipe 14: Homemade glass and window cleaner recipe

Description: Essential oils have the property of protecting the windows from the UV light. The homemade glass and window cleaner spray has such an essential oil which can be successfully used in cleaning your window. Below is the recipe of it.

INGREDIENTS:

- Vinegar- 1/3 cup
- Lavender essential oil- 8 to 9 drops
- A spray bottle
- Water- 2/3 cup

Directions:

- Take your spray bottle and put in the vinegar, the lavender essential oil, and the water and stir and mix it to combine.
- Spray on your window glass, wipe it with a damp towel first and then finally wipe with a dry cloth to remove the stains and clean the glass.
- Store it in a cool place and you can use it any time to clean your window.

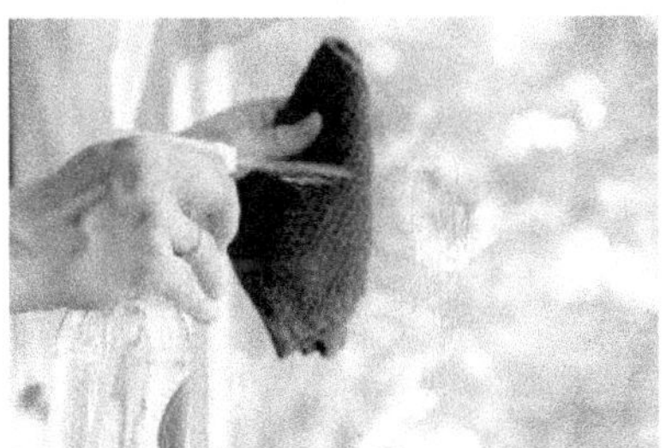

Recipe 15: Fabric refresher

Description: There is a certain kind of smell in some homes and it gets more obvious when we enter our homes. This smell may be in the wardrobes or in the walls, or from the clothes or even the shoes. There is a simple fabric refresher which will make our home smell good and pleasant.

Ingredients:

- Purification essential oil- 5 to 10 drops
- A spray bottle
- Water- 2 to 3 tablespoons

Recipe:

- Take the spray bottle and add in the water and the purification essential oil and mix it well.
- Close the lid and spray it whenever you leave the home, or when you feel it is becoming smelly.
- Whenever you will enter your home you will smell in the pleasant odor.

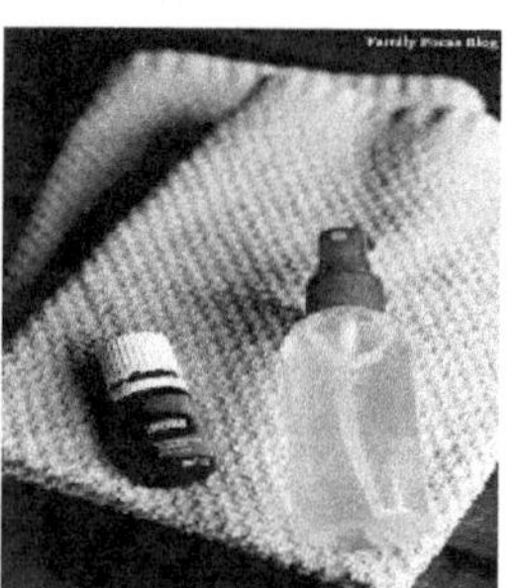

Recipe 16: Homemade bathroom poo spray

Description: If you live in a house with a lot of men around or majority of males there, it must really smell bad in the washroom after one comes out. We have provided you with the recipe of a homemade bathroom poo spray to get rid of the nasty smell in your washroom.

Ingredients:

- Rosemary essential oil- 10 drops
- Lavender essential oil- 20 drops
- Lemon grass essential oil- 10 drops
- A spray bottle
- Vegetable glycerin- 1 Teaspoon
- Water- 1 cup

Directions:

- Combine the rosemary essential oil, the lavender essential oil, the lemongrass essential oil, the water and the vegetable glycerin all together.
- Mix all ingredients well and pour into the spray bottle.
- Close the spray bottle and whenever someone leaves the washroom remind them to spray the bathroom before coming out.
- This way the washroom will not smell bad and whenever you have to go to the washroom it will be having a pleasant smell.

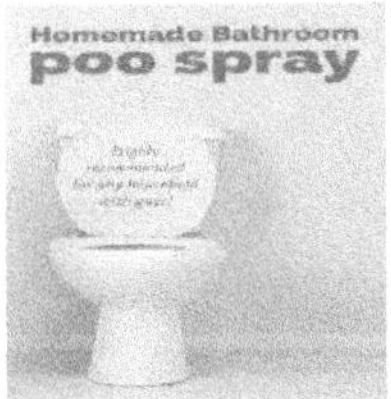

Recipe 17: Homemade dishwasher detergent lab

Description: The detergents available in the grocery store have a lot of chemicals in them. They are full of chemicals. Their use may make our skin to get rough and dry. It is good to replace them with homemade detergents with natural ingredients to get rid of the toxic stuff. Below is a recipe of a homemade dishwasher with essential oil in it.

Ingredients:

- Water- ½ cup
- Citrus fresh essential oil- 45 drops
- Salt- 3 tablespoons
- Nice washing soda- 1 ¼ cups

Directions:

- Take a clean bowl, pour water, washing soda, salt and the citrus essential oil and stir all the ingredients together and mix it well.
- Make sure to mix with a stainless spoon.
- Take a silicon mould and pour the mixture into them and let them cool and set.
- It will take about 48 hours to set completely.
- Keep it in a cool place away from heat.

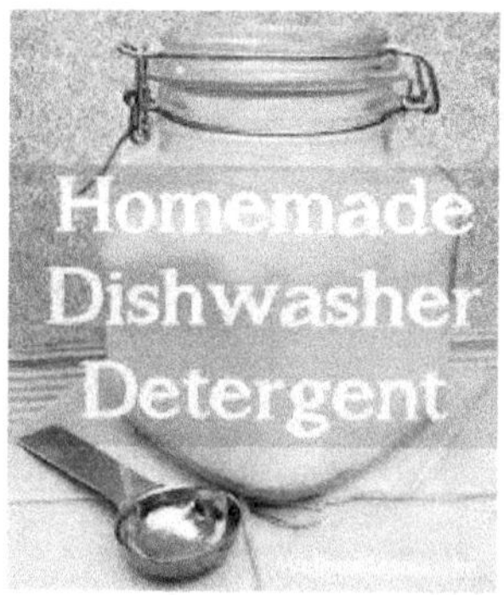

Recipe 18: The perfect shower cleaner recipe

Description: Tired of dirty showers? Use this recipe which makes an excellent shower cleaner and make your showers spotless and clean.

Ingredients:

- Vinegar- ½ cup
- Dish wash liquid- 1 tablespoon
- Tea tree essential oil- 5 drops

Directions:

- Take a spray bottle and add in the vinegar and the dish wash liquid.
- Now add in the tea tree essential oil and shake to mix.
- Spray this on your shower and scrub to clean.
- Your shower is now clean.

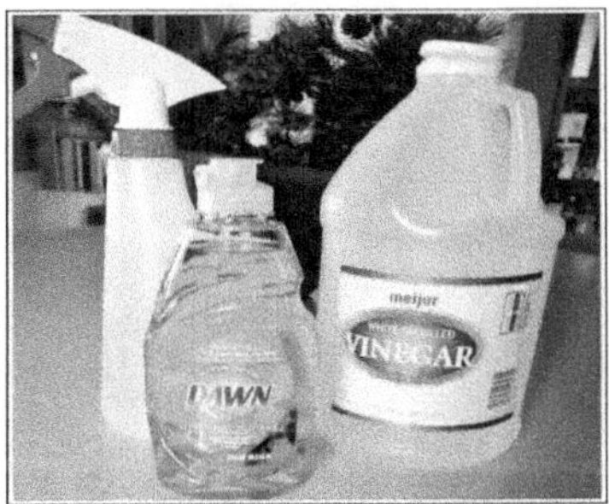

Recipe 19: Window and mirror cleaners

Description: Instead of buying the expensive window and mirror cleaners from the supermarket, try out this amazing recipe in order to achieve the perfect results.

Ingredients:

- Warm water- 2 quarters
- Cornstarch- ½ cup

Directions:

- Take a bowl and mix in the cornstarch with the water.
- Dip a sponge in the liquid and apply it on your mirrors and windows and clean.
- Wipe it with a dry cloth.
- Use a vacuum to completely dry your window.

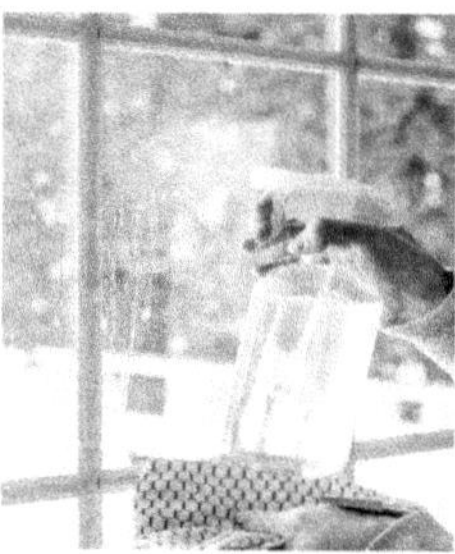

Recipe 20: Homemade glass cleaner recipe

Description: Try out this homemade glass cleaner recipe which makes the use of alcohol to give a great shine to your windows.

Ingredients:

- Isopropyl- 1 cup
- Water- 1 cup
- White vinegar- 1 tablespoon

Directions:

- Take a spray bottle and add in the isopropyl.
- Now mix in the water.
- Stay far when mixing the alcohol with the water as it might cause fumes.
- Now mix in the white vinegar.
- Shake gently to mix in the ingredients.
- Spray on your wall glass or on your window glass and then wipe it off with a damp cloth.

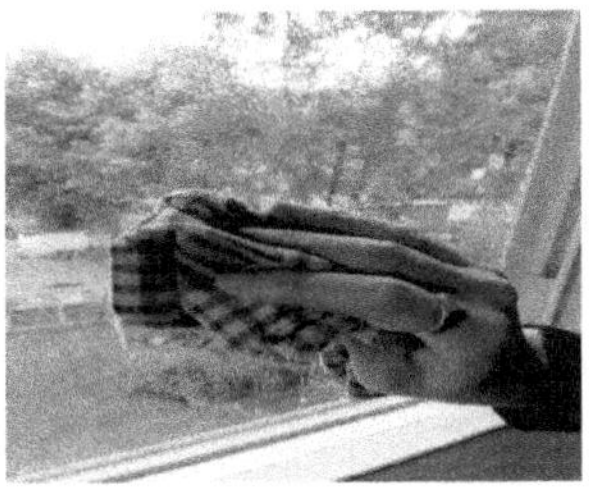

Recipe 21: Extremely strong glass cleaner

Description: In this recipe, ammonia is used which gives a much stronger affect and makes it less difficult to remove the dirt and stains on your glass.

Ingredients:

- Isopropyl alcohol- 1 cup
- Water-1 cup
- Non-sudsing ammonia- 1 tablespoon

Directions:

- Take a spray bottle and add in the isopropyl alcohol.
- Now add in the water and be careful to avoid any kind of mishap.
- Now add in the ammonia and mix well to combine all the ingredients.
- Spray to your desired area which needs to be cleaned and then wipe it off with a cloth.

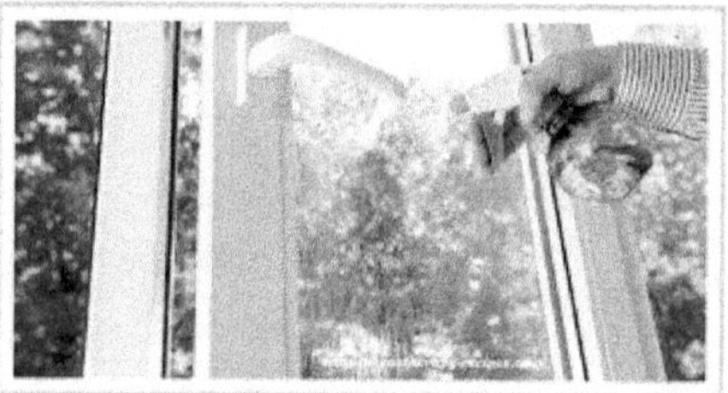

Recipe 22: All-purpose cleaner recipe

Description: Use this all purpose cleaner recipe at your home and stay away from buying the expensive sprays available in the supermarkets.

Ingredients:

- Water- 2 cups
- Dishwashing liquid- 1 tablespoon
- Non sudsing ammonia- 1 tablespoon

Directions:

- Mix together the water, dishwashing liquid and the non sudsing ammonia.
- Shake gently to mix all the ingredients.
- Spray it on any place which you wish to clean.
- Spray and then wipe it off with a damp cloth.

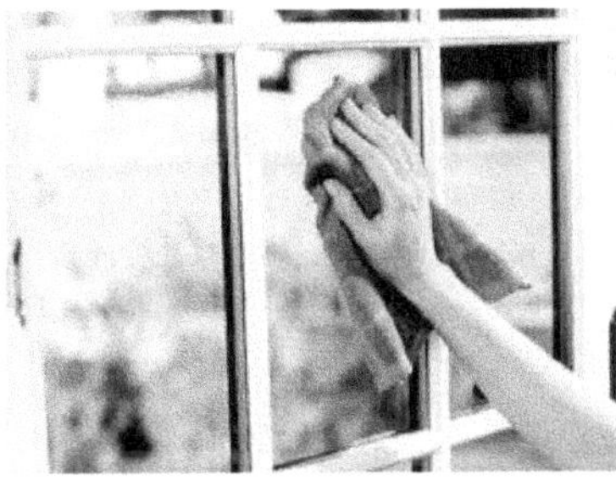

Recipe 23: Kitchen counter cleaner

Description: Kitchen counters tend to get really dirty because all kinds of cutting and chopping is done on them. They are more prone to attract bugs and roaches specially if they are not cleaned properly. Use this recipe of kitchen counter cleaner to have a clean kitchen counter.

Ingredients:

- Baking soda- ½ cup
- Lemon juice- 1/3 cup
- Vinegar- ¼ cup
- Water- 7 cups

Directions:

- Take a spray bottle and mix in the water, vinegar, lemon juice and the baking soda.
- Shake gently so that all the ingredients are mixed properly.
- Spray it on your kitchen counter and then wipe away with a damp cloth to remove all the dirt.

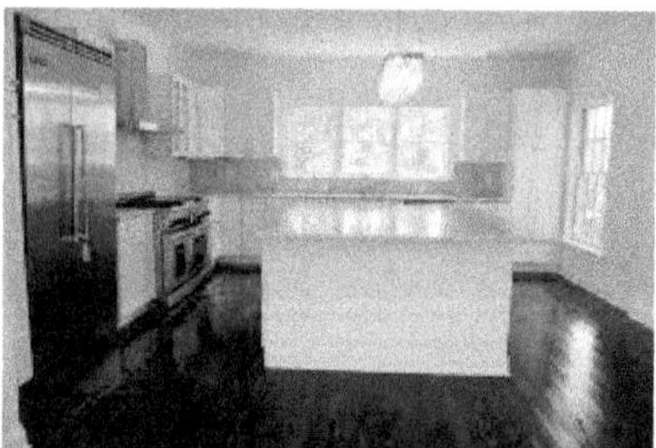

Recipe 24: Microwave cleaner

Description: Microwaves get really smelly because we warm food in them all day. Use this recipe of microwave cleaner to give your microwave a fresh and good scent.

Ingredients:

- White vinegar- ½ cup
- Water- ½ cup

Directions:

- Take a bowl and add in the vinegar and the water and heat the bowl in the microwave for about a minute until it starts boiling.
- Carefully remove the bowl from the microwave and using a paper towel dip it in the bowl once it gets a bit cool and then wipe the interior of your microwave.
- Let the inside dry before closing on your microwave door.
- All smell will be removed by this.

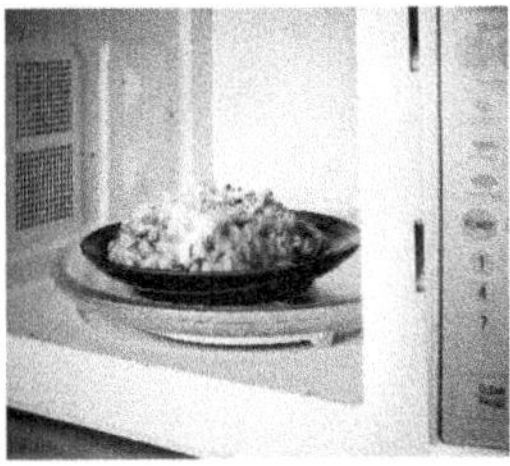

Recipe 25: Toilet scrubber

Description: Toilet bowls can smell nasty and turn dirty in no time. It is important to clean them every day. Use this homemade recipe of a toilet scrubber.

Ingredients:

- White vinegar- 1 cup
- Dish wash liquid- ½ cup

Directions:

- Take a bowl and add in the vinegar and the dish wash liquid.
- Mix together the ingredients and pour in to your toilet bowl and scrub the dirt with the help of a toilet brusher.
- Let it stay for a few hours before flushing.
- Take a bowl and add in the vinegar and the dish wash liquid.
- Mix together the ingredients and pour in to your toilet bowl and scrub the dirt with the help of a toilet brusher.
- Let it stay for a few hours before flushing.

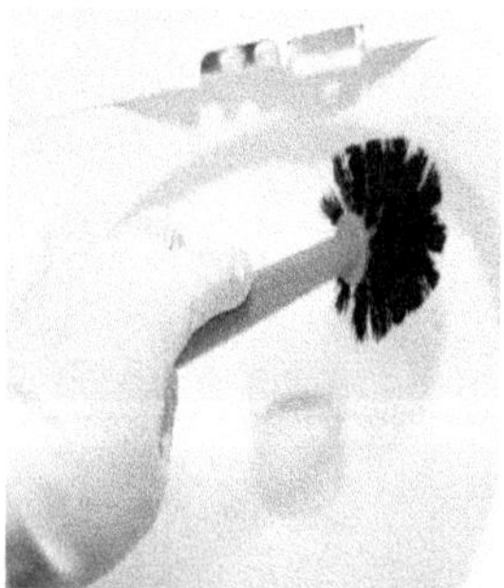

Recipe 26: Kitchen counter top cleaner

Description: Use this excellent homemade kitchen counter cleaner recipe to clean and wipe away the dirt from your kitchen counters

Ingredients:

- Baking soda- 1 2/3 cup
- Liquid soap- ½ cup
- Water- ½ cup
- Vinegar- 2 tablespoons

Directions:

- Add the water in the bowl and then mix in the baking soda.
- Now add in the liquid soap and the vinegar.
- Mix together all the ingredients.
- Using a damp towel clean your kitchen counters with this mixture and then wipe away with a dry towel.

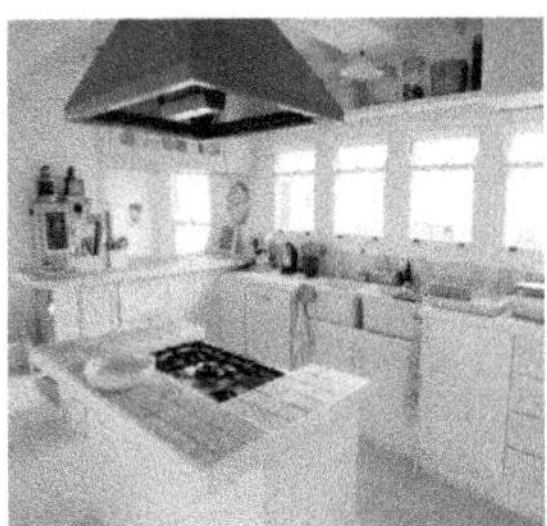

Recipe 27: How to remove water stains from kitchen counters

Description: Water stains are common on kitchen counters specially if you keep wet dishes or glasses on the counters. You can use this recipe to get rid of water stains.

Ingredients:

- Non-gel toothpaste- 2 tablespoons
- Baking soda- 2 tablespoons

Directions:

- Mix together the non-gel tooth paste and the baking soda.
- With the help of a cloth rub on to the counters and then wipe it away with a damp towel.
- Repeat this process every day for a few days until the stains disappear.

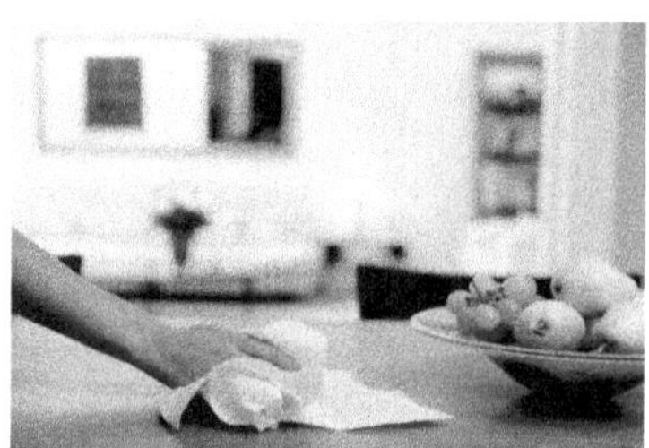

Recipe 28: How to remove rust from kitchen counter tops and on taps

Description: Rusting is very common and it disrupts the entire show of your kitchen or any place where it erupts. Follow this tip below to learn how to deal with rusting.

Ingredients:

- Lemon- ½
- Salt- 1 tablespoon

Directions:

- Cut your lemon in to half.
- Dip one half of your lemon in to the salt.
- Rub this dipped lemon on the rusty area.
- Let it stand for a while before washing it with water or cleaning with a damp towel.

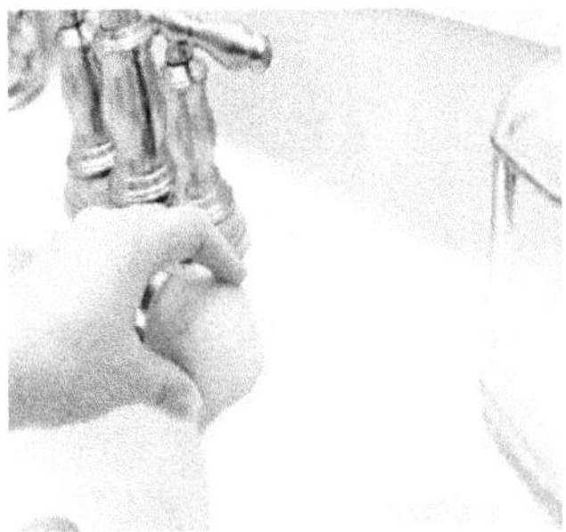

Recipe 29: How to sparkle and shine your bathtub

Description: Here is an excellent way to make your bathtub shine and sparkle by making this simple spray at home.

Ingredients:

- Water- to fill your tub
- Oxygen bleach- 1 scoop

Directions:

- Close the lid of your bath tub and fill it completely with water.
- Now add in the scoop of oxygen bleach.
- Let the water stay like this for the night.
- Discard the water the next day and check out the shine of your bath tub.

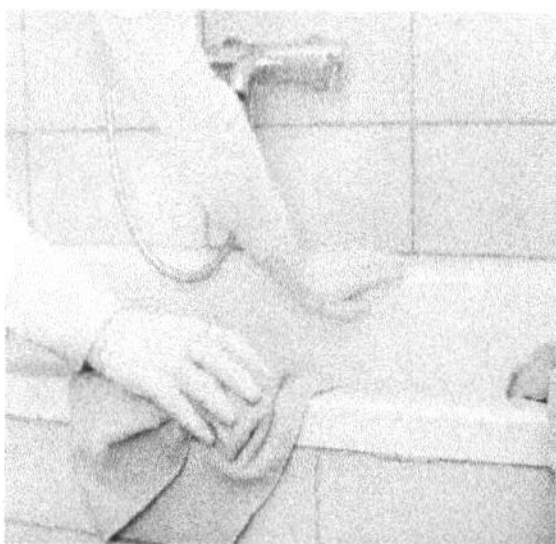

Recipe 30: How to shine water taps

Description: Water taps tend to get blurred, dirty and rusty. Use the following tip to get sparkling taps.

Ingredients:

- Cotton ball- 1
- Baby oil- 1 tablespoon

Directions:

- Using a cotton ball dip in to the baby oil.
- Polish it on your faucet or tap and then wash it with water.
- Dry it with a towel and you will see it perfectly shining and gleaming.

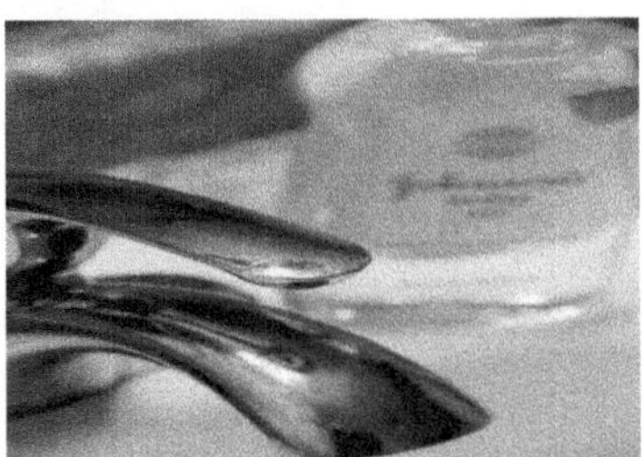

Recipe 31: How to remove rust stains from basins and surfaces

Description: Use this simple recipe to remove all kinds of stains and rusts from your basins and surfaces and make them shine like they are new again.

Ingredients:

- Cream of tartar- 1 tablespoon
- Lemon juice- 1

Directions:

- Make a mixture by mixing together the juice of one lemon and the cream of tartar.
- Dip any old toothbrush in to the mixture and then dab it on the surface or your basin to remove the rust.

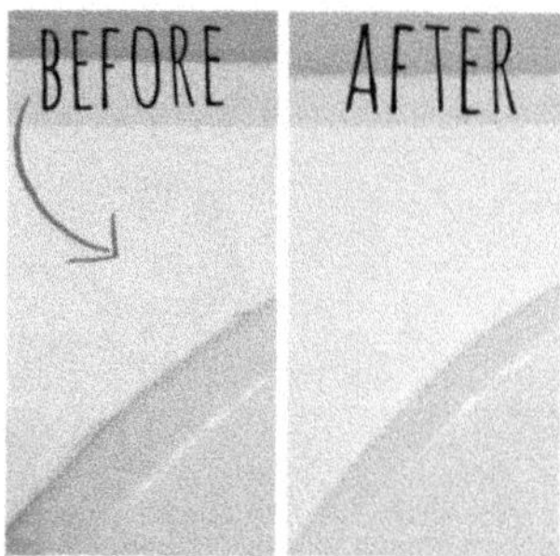

Recipe 32: How to clean kitchen granite countertops

Description: Every material has a different method of cleaning and so granite kitchen counter tops are cleaned differently too. Use this recipe to find out how to clean kitchen granite counter tops.

Ingredients:

- Water-2 cups
- Rubbing alcohol- ¼ cup
- Dishwashing liquid- 4 to 5 drops

Directions:

- Mix together the water, alcohol and the dishwashing liquid.
- Apply this mixture through a wet cloth on your granite kitchen counter.
- Wipe away with a dry cloth.

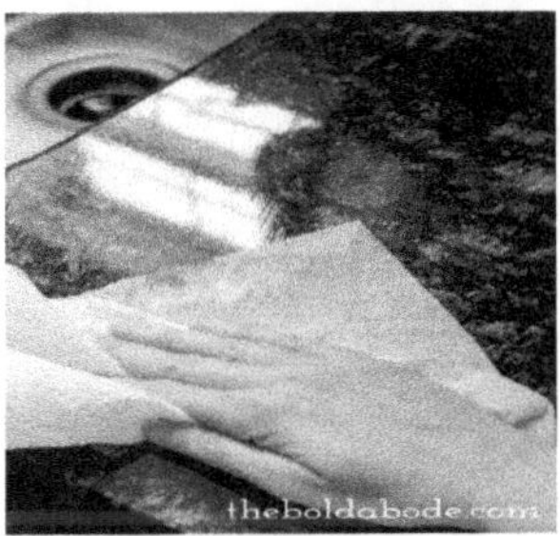

Recipe 33: How to clean your kitchen sink

Description: Use the following recipe to clean your kitchen sink and make it spotlessly clean with just a few ingredients.

Ingredients:

- Baking soda- 1 teaspoon
- Hydrogen peroxide- 2 teaspoon

Directions:

- Mix together the baking soda and the hydrogen peroxide.
- Take a damp towel and dip in the mixed mixture.
- Clean your basin with this towel and let it stay like this for 2 hours.
- Wash your basin now to see your reflection smiling back at you.

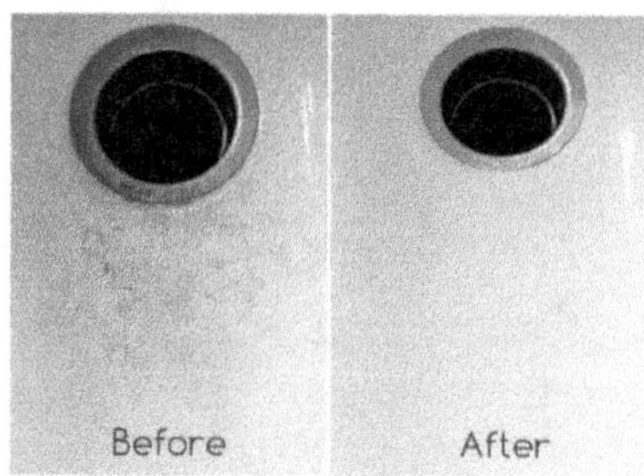

Recipe 34: How to clean your baking oven

Description: Use the following recipe to clean your baking ovens as they tend to get dirty and germs also accumulate inside.

Ingredients:

- Baking soda- 1 cup
- Liquid dish soap- 1 tablespoon
- Water- 1 tablespoon

Directions:

- Make a paste by mixing in the following ingredients baking soda, liquid dish soap and the water.
- Dip a damp towel inside and put in on your oven and let sit for 15 minutes.
- Wipe it away and see the results almost instantly!

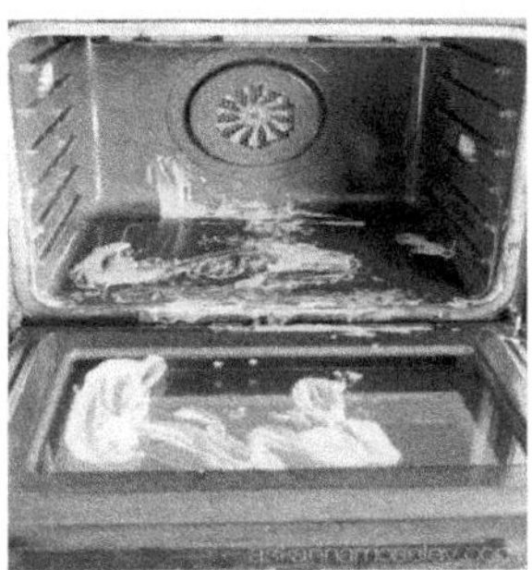

Recipe 35: How to clean stove burners

Description: All day cooking makes the stove burners to be really dirty. It is best if this recipe is followed and so you can clean your burners easily with this tip.

Ingredients:

- Baking soda- 1 tablespoon
- Dish wash liquid- 2 tablespoons

Directions:

- Take a bowl and mix the baking soda and the dish wash liquid to make a thick paste.
- Using damp towel clean your stove burners with this mixture and then dry it with a cloth.
- You will get great results!

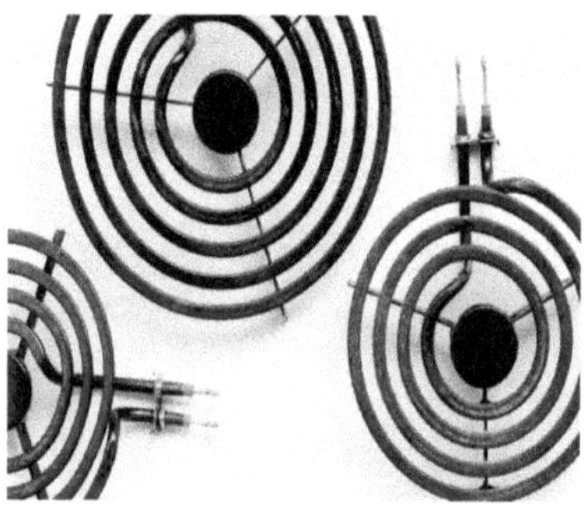

Recipe 36: How to clean your gas stove

Description: Using this recipe you can very easily clean your gas stove and even remove the rusts from it.

Ingredients:

- Baking soda- 1 tablespoon
- Hydrogen peroxide- 1 tablespoon
- Tea tree essential oil- 5 drops

Directions:

- Take a bowl and add in the baking soda, hydrogen peroxide and the tea tree essential oil.
- Apply this on your stove and then wipe it away with a damp towel.
- Your oven will be perfectly clean.

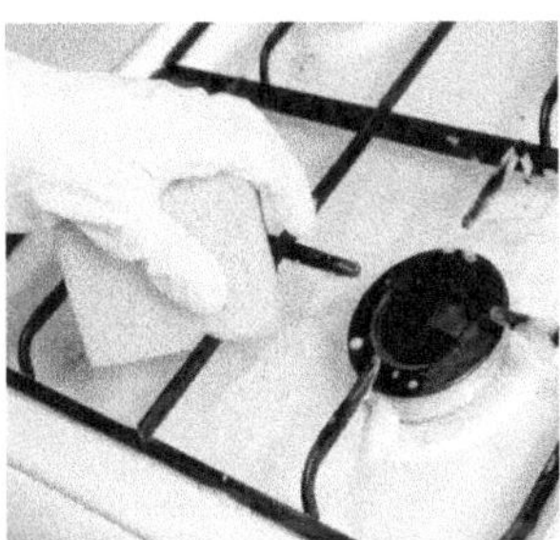

Recipe 37: How to clean your oven door

Description: Clean your oven door using this tip as this homemade tip can be easily made and it is very affective in cleaning your oven door as well.

Ingredients:

- Baking soda- 1 teaspoon
- Soap bar- ½
- Water- 1 cup

Directions:

- Soak your soap bar in the water until it turns in to a soapy water.
- Sprinkle baking soda on your oven door and then using a damp cloth clean your oven door with the soapy water.
- Leave it to stay for 15 minutes before wiping it off properly.

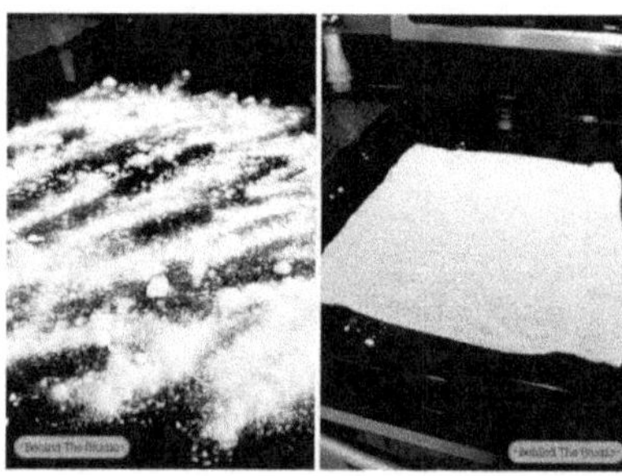

Recipe 38: How to wash windows

Description: This is a very unique tip about cleaning windows using simply onion and it will make your windows to shine perfectly.

Ingredients:

- Onion- 1, cut in to half

Directions:

- Cut your onion in half and simply rub it on your window glass.
- Let it stay for a while like this.
- Take a damp cloth and rub it over the window glass.
- Your window glass is now clean.

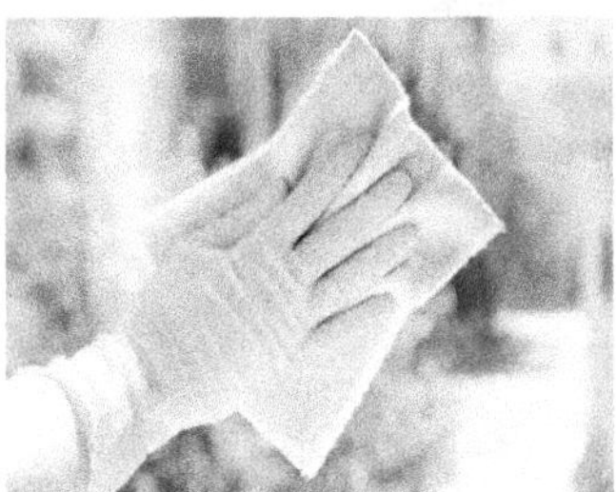

Recipe 39: How to shine your tiles

Description: Use this tip to clean your floors and tiles instead of buying expensive floor cleaners. Here is the recipe.

Ingredients:

- Soap- a bar
- Hydrogen peroxide- 5 drops
- Water- 1 cup

Directions:

- Soak the soap bar in to water until the water gets soapy.
- Strain and fill this soapy water in to a spray bottle.
- Now add in the hydrogen peroxide and give it a shake.
- Mix properly.
- Spray it on your tile and then wipe it away with a damp cloth.
- Your tiles will shine perfectly.

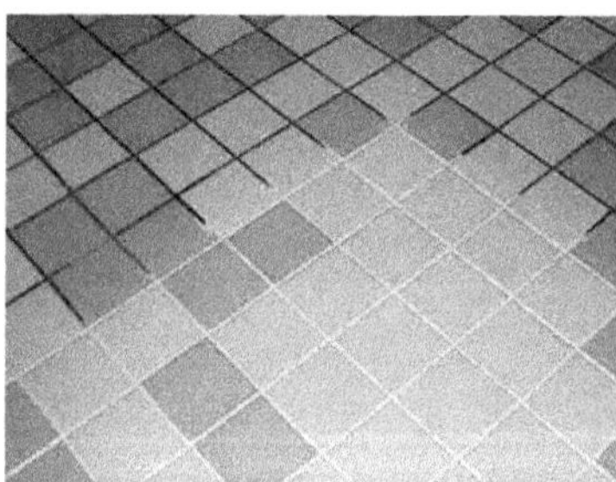

Recipe 40: How to clean marble kitchen counter tops

Description: Kitchen counter tops are made of different materials. Some are of granite while some are of marble. Each has its own way and method of cleaning. Below is the recipe to clean your marble kitchen counter tops.

Ingredients:

- Marble polishing powder- 3 tablespoons

Directions:

- First of all, wet your kitchen counter top by the help of a water spray bottle.
- After that, sprinkle on with some marble polishing powder.
- Use a damp towel and wipe away the powder.
- Your kitchen marble counter top will now shine.

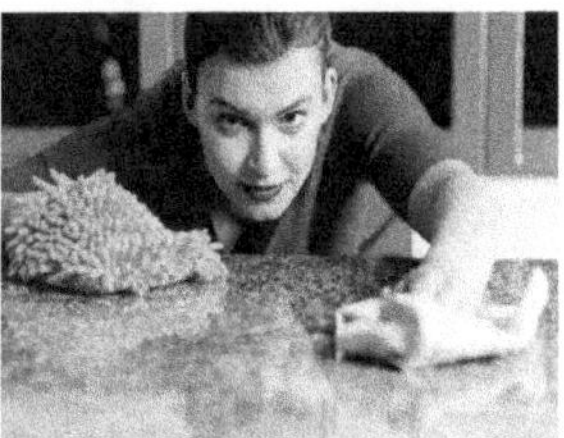

Conclusion

The following book, Homemade Household Cleaners: 40 Recipes of Safe Cleaners for Tiles, Stoves, Ovens And Kitchen Countertops is a great read for those who want to follow successful tips in order to get rid of rusts, stains, greases and dirt from their tiles, counter tops, ovens and burners.

This book tells you 40 such tips which you can follow easily at your home and then benefit yourselves.

The safety cleaners that are available out there in the supermarkets are not only expensive but they are also stuffed with dangerous chemicals some of which have known to cause deadly diseases such as cancer.

Other common problems include asthma and migraines both of which are very problematic. It is advised therefore, that you should give upon those readily made safety cleaners and opt for the homemade ones.

These homemade safety cleaners are not only chemical free but they are also very easy to make. You can easily make these at home using just a few simple ingredients that are normally available at your home.

However, it is advised that you should be very careful and keep away these cleaners from children specially crawling babies as they can be harmful to their health if mistakenly eaten.

The mixing of alcohol with water should be done very carefully as it can cause fumes to erupt and that can be dangerous. It is advisable to wear protective gloves and goggles while making these safety cleaners at home. It is best that you prepare these safety cleaners in a very careful manner so as to avoid any mishap.

When you are done with making your safety cleaners, use a permanent marker and a stick on to stick on the respective bottle and then label it with the type of safety cleaner it is so you can save it for later use. It is also advised not to use fizzy drink or juice bottles for this purpose as this can be really deceiving for small children. The best thing to do is to keep these safety cleaner bottles and sprays on a great height where small hands cannot reach out to grasp them.

Get this book as fast as you can and learn these 40 safety cleaner tips and shine your house without having any trouble!

FREE Bonus Reminder

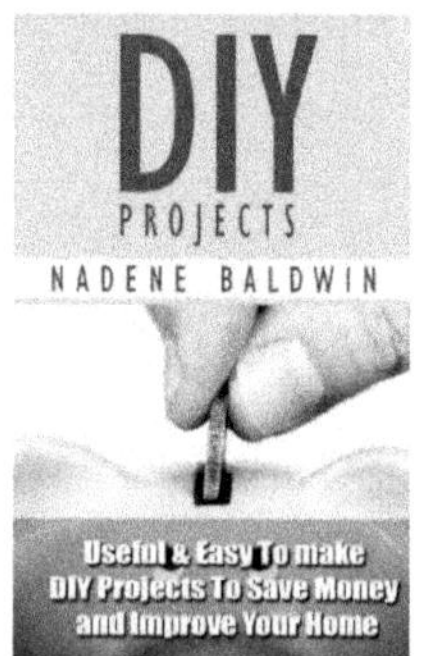

If you have not grabbed it yet, please go ahead and download your special bonus report *"DIY Projects. 13 Useful & Easy To Make DIY Projects To Save Money & Improve Your Home!"*
Simply Click the Button Below

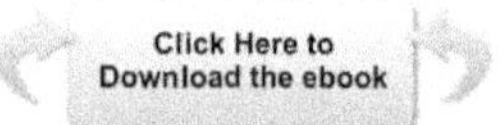

OR **Go to This Page**
http://diyhomecraft.com/free

BONUS #2: More Free & Discounted Books or Products
Do you want to receive more Free/Discounted Books or Products?
We have a mailing list where we send out our new Books or Products when they go free or with a discount on Amazon. Click on the link below to sign up for Free & Discount Book & Product Promotions.
=> Sign Up for Free & Discount Book & Product Promotions <=

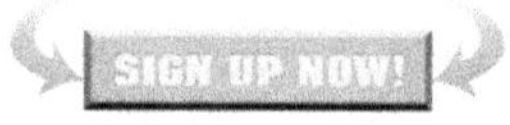

OR Go to this URL
http://bit.ly/1WBb1Ek